Drug Free Holist

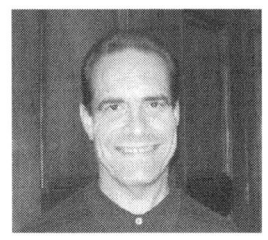

Drug-Free Holistic Approach to Parkinson's Disease

> **How long has it been since you fully recovered from Parkinson's disease?**

HOWARD SHIFKE: June 12th (2010) is the last time that I had any Parkinson's symptoms. The symptoms had started the previous September, the ones that were recognizable to me. In August 2010, a couple of months after realizing that I no longer had symptoms, it was time for my six-month follow up visit with my neurologist. He exclaimed at the end of our visit after putting me through all of his tests that he was unable to detect a single Parkinson's symptom as well.

> **Are you symptom-free today?**

HOWARD SHIFKE: I have been

© *Parkinsons Recovery*

Drug Free Holistic Approach

completely symptom-free since June 12th of 2010.

> **When did you realize you might have Parkinson's and what did you do in response to that realization?**

HOWARD SHIFKE: In September of 2009 I was sitting at my desk doing some work and I started to feel like my entire body was shaking. I looked down at my arms, which were then on the armrests of my chair and I noticed that there was no movement at all; however, I felt this tremendous tremoring inside. So being as I was sitting at my desk at my computer, I opened up Google and typed in 'internal tremors.' Everything that came up was related to Parkinson's disease.

I started first thinking, well, this can't be right. My mother had Parkinson's disease and she passed away in February of 2007. Parkinson's was a little bit in the back of my mind, but it certainly was not in the foreground at the time. I went from article

Drug Free Holistic Approach

to article reviewing specifically what authors of various articles were saying the symptoms of Parkinson's disease were. Of course as I read an article and reviewed the symptoms that were listed, I would reflect a bit and realize I had the same symptoms. I'd then say to myself, "Well, this article must be incorrect." So, article after article after article of what I felt were probably incorrect people, I reached one that not only had listed the main symptoms but also listed what they considered to be smaller or lesser known potential symptoms. It was a list of about 15 items. I had to be honest with myself as I went down that list, I realized at some level I had everything that was on it and that was my greatest realization at that moment. At that point in time, I decided to wait a day to see if everything I was experiencing at that moment would go away. It did not. So the following day I knew I had to sit down with my wife and talk about it with her.

Drug Free Holistic Approach

> **What careers have you had?**

HOWARD SHIFKE: I had practiced law from 1986 until 1999 and then from 1999 until present I've been involved in sales and marketing of technology products, software and hardware and primarily software in the healthcare field.

> **Why did you decide to take a holistic approach?**

HOWARD SHIFKE: I guess this is kind of the longer part of the beginning of the story. There are a few reasons. One of the reasons was having watched my mother over the course of 24 years with Parkinson's disease. She went through what was the way of being diagnosed with Parkinson's at the time. That began with misdiagnosis and medications for the things that might have been Parkinson's but were not. Ultimately when she did not get better or feel better in any way, she then was put on the Parkinson's medications which, compared to how she

Drug Free Holistic Approach

had been feeling for those previous years of treatment, made her feel better. She received the Parkinson's diagnosis and was on the Parkinson's medications for 20 plus years. Over a couple of decades, ultimately the medications and the disease took their toll on her. It was not a very pretty ending. It was rather sad because she also ended up suffering from a level of Alzheimer's and Dementia and as you know, that is a very hard way to see somebody prior to their death with Parkinson's and Alzheimer's and Dementia. I had that fairly fresh in my mind.

For years I had just taken a liking to and studied through books and articles, traditional Chinese medicines and alternative healing and holistic healing and there were many things that we had done around here as a family over the years that gave me a very strong belief and feeling that alternative or holistic approaches to fighting maladies could end

Drug Free Holistic Approach

in great success.

And of course as you know, Parkinson's is designated as an incurable disease. Although the medications may help with pain or they may help with mobility, they do not lead toward recovery and they do not lead toward a cure. This is not just me talking about that, but I think that it's fairly common knowledge that there's a greater level of comfort that one may have in taking the medications but ultimately, there is not an expectation in taking the medications or an expectation when the medications are prescribed that the individual is going to improve, recover or be cured.

There has been nearly 200 years of information since James Parkinson discovered the disease. It seemed to me that I needed to put my faith in the holistic approach and at least get started going down that path. The other path in the background may be an alternative, but

Drug Free Holistic Approach

having seen the potential of how it could end with my mother, I felt a very strong need to go in a different direction and to go on a different path.

I had the full support of my wife with that decision and in a large way I felt I owed it to my wife and our three children to try to fight the disease rather than accept the disease and where I might go if I was taking the medications. When I say "in fighting the disease," I had read an article early on that the author said that when people receive a diagnosis of cancer that he had seen that they take a hard line, "I'm going to fight this" approach, and that when people receive a diagnosis of Parkinson's, it is an acceptance of an inevitable end. I was not in denial that I had Parkinson's, but I was definitely denying that there wasn't a different way to approach it.

Drug Free Holistic Approach

> **Before your diagnosis of Parkinson's disease had you personally experienced various holistic approaches?**

HOWARD SHIFKE: Yes. Yes. That was part of what gave me confidence that at least I could give it a good fight. And from doing Qigong exercises to Jin Shin Jyutsu to energy work, acupressure, there are certain things that we had learned. If one of my children caught a cold or had a runny nose or something of that nature, there is a certain acupressure that we would do that would open up the sinuses and drain the cold. Within a couple of days without having to be on any medications, we would get rid of a basic cold.

We're not talking about things at the level of a major disease like Parkinson's or any other major disease, but sure, things like a cold or if somebody had a pain, then there was certain acupressure or a certain Qigong exercise or a certain way of doing

Drug Free Holistic Approach

energy work where we would handle the pain.

I think part of what we learned along the way in doing it is a little bit of a different mindset. And when I say a little bit of a different mindset, when one of us would have a cold or have a pain or have a health issue, we would sit down and look at it not from the "what is the symptom," but from "what may have caused the symptom?" In the books I have on traditional Chinese medicine, it's very helpful in going through because in treating the individual as a total organism as opposed to just treating where a certain pain might be, I feel we were very successful. Nothing was really major, but over the years we were very successful in treating small health issues around the house by getting to the heart of the matter of what may have caused it and then dealing with the cause rather than just dealing with getting rid of the pain.

Drug Free Holistic Approach

> **When did you see a neurologist and receive a diagnosis of Parkinson's disease?**

HOWARD SHIFKE: I scheduled an appointment and saw my neurologist November 5th of 2009, which was about five weeks after I started getting the tremors and realized that I probably did have Parkinson's disease. When I went to the neurologist, he put me through all of his tests and he did confirm the diagnosis. Obviously there is always that hope, I mean I pretty much knew I had it, but there's always that hope that you go and the neurologist says no, you don't have it, but I kind of knew what the diagnosis would be and I received the diagnosis that I did in fact have Parkinson's.

> **Give us a brief preview of your visit to the neurologist**

HOWARD SHIFKE: First we sat down and had a lengthy discussion of why I was there. There had been times earlier in the year when I had experienced some health

Drug Free Holistic Approach

issues that were significant enough to me that I notated them, just for paying attention purposes. I was able to give at least accurate information and general dates and times relative to things that were happening. I was able to explain to him that in February of 2009, I was at the gas station and when I went to pump the gas, I could not squeeze the pump. I realized that I had really bad pain on the outer part of the muscle near my elbow. Then I realized shortly after that that I was unable to lift the water pitcher with my left arm because of the same pain and the inability to actually grasp the handle. As denial will go, back in November 2009, I thought well, I probably just hurt my arm; let me not use it. So I just started using my right hand for everything. I was at least able to tell him that along the way, the pain never subsided.

I did have a sense of slowness. I recalled over a course of months that I would be walking along or going up the stairs in the

Drug Free Holistic Approach

house and think, "If this is how I feel at 48 years of age, I cannot imagine how I'm going to feel 20 years from now because I'm feeling kind of slow, old and painful." These are the little type of recognitions that I had.

A substantial part of the tests that he gave me were movement tests. I did walking and balance tests. He did tests with my eye movements. While sitting on the table he would have me tap on my right side with my right hand while holding my left arm straight out in front. At first my left arm froze and then it got a mind all of its own and started, for lack of a better word, flailing all over the place.

Then he switched that up. I remember that I was tapping my left side with my left palm and had my right arm out and experienced the same thing but really to a fraction of a degree of what had gone on with my other side. My right arm got very tight and moved around quite a bit. I

Drug Free Holistic Approach

could not hold it steady at all and could not stop it from moving, but my right arm did not have nearly as much flailing that my left arm had shown. Those are the main tests that I remember. There were other physical tests that compared left-side versus right side movements which included balance tests and walking tests.

> **What did you learn from doing these tests at the neurologist's office?**

HOWARD SHIFKE: Thank you for asking that. This actually for me was one of the greatest learning experiences that I think helped in a huge way in my recovery. That is, I learned that the left side of my body and the right side of my body were not talking to each other. They weren't working well. The wires were crossed. If I was going to continue to try to recover then I needed to figure a way to isolate the right side of my body and isolate the left side of my body so that I would be able to function better.

Drug Free Holistic Approach

The left side of the brain operates the right side of the body and the right side of the brain operates the left side of the body. They say with Parkinson's, by the time you start to have the really big symptoms, the kind that make you go to a neurologist - that upwards of 60% to 80% of the basal ganglia in the brain controlling your movement are dead. So it made me realize that theoretically, if I was working with only 20% to 40% of the neural impulses controlling my movement, I needed to streamline the electricity in a better way. I felt that I needed to learn exactly what was going on inside my body so that I would have a better opportunity to try to fix it.

I decided I needed to see where the neural impulses went because obviously from the tests that the doctor gave me, movement on one side of the body set off uncontrollable reactions on the other side of the body. I started a process in the morning where I would stand in the

Drug Free Holistic Approach

kitchen, hold on to the counter with one hand and while I was doing this, slowly lift my other hand out to side. I had terrible balance. My balance was somewhere behind my heels, so I really needed to hunch forward in order to stay upright. What I would do is stand there, hold the counter with my left hand and I would take my right arm, have it hang down by my side and then I would lift it straight out to the side, slowly. I would do that four times and then I would close my eyes and see what I felt.

When I first started doing this I would notice that I had very strong electrical impulses sometimes in my left knee or my left shoulder, even though it had been my right arm that I was moving. So I went online and I found the outline of a body. I printed it up and made a bunch of copies and so I started working on trying to isolate where the neural impulses were in my body in response to moving each limb one at a time. I'd do the right arm, then

Drug Free Holistic Approach

the left arm. Then I would do one leg and then the other. With the legs, I would just bring it up as much as I could in what I would say like a marching position; you just bring it up and put it down four times and then see where I felt the impulses. Through that process, I started to learn a little bit more about what was going on electrically inside my body.

I started to do things 'one-sided' so that I had to really focus. The best example I could give is that I generally drove the car left-handed and with my right foot on the pedals. It occurred to me that if I have, after extended driving some type of a freezing or non-controlling movement in my left arm as a result of moving my right foot, or in my right foot as a result of moving my left arm. This could result in a terrible accident when driving the car.

So, I changed my method of driving. I started putting my left hand under my left thigh so that I took it completely out of

Drug Free Holistic Approach

the equation. I learned how to drive just with my right hand so that all of my movement was on that one side of my body. This is where I was fortunate that I had years of experience of reading and doing and a number of holistic things because I remembered that I had read about a 'brain-vibration chant.'

Zhi Gang Sha is a Chinese medical doctor and also a western medical doctor. Dr. Sha has an approach called 'soul-mind-body medicine.' Part of his approach involves chanting. The chanting is actually vibrating different parts of your body. I found the brain vibrations chant in one of my books and started doing it to stimulate activity in my brain. I then focused and visualized streamlining the electrical impulses in my body. My goal was to re-train my brain so that the right side of my brain would move the right side of my body and the left side of my brain would move the left side of my body. I figured that if I could achieve that then I

Drug Free Holistic Approach

would have a much more streamlined approach to my movement. I would take out of the equation the issue of freezing or uncontrolled movement because there would be no cross-over.

I worked on that a lot and that's why I appreciate the question. It was something that I really did not realize until being put through the test what a violent reaction my body had when trying to move left side and right side at the same time.

> **How does the brain chant help to offer relief from symptoms?**

HOWARD SHIFKE: *Dr. Sha shares a lot of information and videos on his* website *and has written a number of books. The first book that I had ever got by Dr. Sha was called* Power Healing. *It's in that book that he first discusses it. In* Soul, Mind, Body Medicine *he talks about the brain-vibration chanting as well.*

Dr. Guo who is Dr. Sha's teacher and mentor and also a Chinese medical doctor

Drug Free Holistic Approach

in China, learned through meditation and trial and error that in Mandarin Chinese saying numbers out loud could create certain vibrations in the body. Through practice, he was able to discover that certain combinations of the numbers could lead to vibrations of the organs or vibrations of your limbs so that it could lead to healing. The idea behind the healing is that the cause of what is wrong with the individual either has to do with too much energy or too little energy. By putting the <u>chanting</u> into the equation, you're creating a vibration that either increases the energy or helps dissipate the energy, depending upon what malady you have.

What does the chanting sound like?

HOWARD SHIFKE: The English phonetic sounds for the brain-vibration chant are: ling, yow, che-che-che, joe, ling, ba; ling, yow, chee-chee-chee, joe, ar, ar, sih, sih (like "sit" without the "t"). This is a unique combination of numbers in

Drug Free Holistic Approach

Chinese. When doing the chant, I would sit forward in a chair as straight up as I could. When I first started doing the chant I actually typed it up and put it on the computer screen so I could stare at it. The idea is that you chant that sequence for say five minutes as fast as possible. It will create a vibration that stimulates the neural impulses in your brain.

How often did you do the chanting?

HOWARD SHIFKE: I did five minutes in the morning, afternoon and the evening. I would feel neural impulses and a lot of activity going on particularly in the back part of my head. I would visualize what was going on in my head; visualize the energy on the right side of my brain going down the right side of my body and the energy in my left side of my brain going down the left side of my body. I was using the brain activity that I was creating through the chanting to visualize and re-train my brain to streamline where the impulses were going.

© *Parkinsons Recovery*

Drug Free Holistic Approach

> Why did you believe that your body could heal itself?

HOWARD SHIFKE: A big part of that belief comes from the experience of the previous years where we had worked on helping our children heal as I explained earlier. If you break it down to the nuts and bolts, I think everybody at some point in their life has experienced natural healing at some level – even if they are not really aware of thinking of it in terms of the body healing itself.

Consider a simple example. You are ten years old. You fall out of the tree and break your arm. Your Mom takes you to the doctor and the doctor says, "Hey, Robert, no big deal. I'm going to set your arm, I'm going to put it in the cast and after x-amount of time you're going to come back here and it is going to be good as new. It might even be better because sometimes when there's a break, it will be stronger than it was before when it is healed."

Drug Free Holistic Approach

Think about the healing process that is involved here. The doctor sets the arm and puts it in a cast, but essentially the body is what heals the arm. Yes, it does take the doctor's expertise in knowing how to properly set the arm and do all of that. The doctor is a very critical part of the formula. But ultimately, what goes on inside the arm - inside the cast - is your body doing the work of healing itself. I am just a strong believer that if you listen to your body and try to make sense of what it is telling you, then you can put things into place that will help your body heal itself.

> **Why should someone "listen to their body" and take a "less-is-more" approach to healing?**

HOWARD SHIFKE: Within a few days of the tremors starting, I had three major limitations that came upon me.

I could not get out of a chair without holding on to the arms of the chair and using my upper body to literally lift me out of a chair.

Drug Free Holistic Approach

No matter how hard I tried I could not convince either of my feet to step on the first step of our stairs unless I first grabbed onto the railing. I reached, I walked up to the stairs one day and that was it. My body stopped right there.

In the middle of eating one day I lifted the food with my utensil and that's where it stopped. I couldn't figure out how to get the utensil with the food to my mouth. I had to concentrate on moving the utensil to my mouth. The result was almost like a cogwheel motion, click-click-click-click-click-click-click-click, about eight clicks at the elbow to get it to my mouth. That was very, very difficult.

I then also realized my arms didn't swing. The rigidity that I had in my back was probably the most painful part of the disease. It made me hunch forward, pulled my shoulders in and really just hurt all the time. Not taking any medications or any supplements or anything to deal

Drug Free Holistic Approach

with the pain allowed me the opportunity to pay attention to where I had the pain so I could figure why I had the pain.

Actually it all started to make pretty good sense. My balance as I mentioned earlier was really terrible. I might get two or three steps and then head backwards head-first to the tile floor which would have been a complete disaster. Same thing with getting out of a chair; if I stood up too quickly and tried to walk, that would have resulted in a similar outcome: head backwards to the floor. I really don't have anything to offer great about the challenge I faced with eating except maybe I was eating too much. I had the darnedest time getting the food to my mouth so I really had a hard time making sense of that one.

I can tell you that I never fell in the nine months that I was actively fighting this disease – I never fell. I never had a hard freezing moment in the middle of walking.

Drug Free Holistic Approach

Part of it, which made sense particularly after my doctor visit, is that my arms had stopped swinging. I didn't know how long prior to realizing I had the disease that my arms had stopped swinging or that I was hunched over or that I was shuffling my feet. It had been some time.

By looking at those limitations I feel that in a way, it was like my body was protecting itself from falling. I was protected from freezing. I would imagine if I had tried to forcibly swing my arms at some point in time, one of my legs would have frozen or have gone out of control and maybe I would have fallen. This is all no different than the tests that my neurologist was running. So, I worked at trying to pay much more attention to those things.

One of the things that anybody who has Parkinson's can tell you is that it really wears you out physically. In a way it's a little bit difficult to explain the issue of

Drug Free Holistic Approach

rigidity. The best way that I've found to explain rigidity is to imagine you're flexing your muscles and then trying to do regular movements with your muscles flexed all day. It's going to wear you out and it's going to hurt after a while.

In order to try to move a little bit better and have a little bit more energy at the end of the day, my "less-is-more approach" to fighting the disease was basically that I didn't push my physical limits to what Parkinson's would allow me to do. I actually stopped prior to that. I walked a little bit slower than Parkinson's would allow me.

I realized that when I would go up the stairs in the conventional manner (where you go every-other step with your feet walking up) that I was having to use a large amount of upper body energy and strength. I was primarily pulling myself up because every time I picked up a foot to go to the next step my body wanted to go

Drug Free Holistic Approach

backwards. It was a physical battle to go up the stairs.

I took a different approach. I decided that instead of going every other step, I would hold on to the railing, put my foot on the first step and then just bring the other foot up to the same step. It was a slower process. Over time it was much easier and barely took any energy at all. If the railing was on my left side and I held on to the railing with my left hand, once I would put my one foot on the step, just by straightening out that knee, the other foot would come up to the step next to it. Movement was slower but I could stand a little straighter when I walked and I could go up and down the stairs, albeit it took me longer. I could do it without a lot of physical exertion.

I started to really pay attention to what "my body was telling me." When I say 'paying attention,' I took the attitude when something would happen that I didn't like because it was another physical thing that I couldn't do any more, I would stop, think about it and say, "Well, let's try to make some sense of it." More times than not I was able to at least justify or make some sense of the limitation. I would then try to approach my physical movement from a slower direction or slower way of moving than I had before in order to, as I would say, best respond to my body telling me, "Don't do these things."

Did you take any medications?

HOWARD SHIFKE: I did not. I did not for a couple of reasons. One of them is that once I came to the conclusion that I really needed to listen to my body if I was going to have any chance of recovering from this disease. I did not want to take anything that would mask a symptom. I did not want to take any medicine that might give me better movement than maybe I was supposed to have with the disease, or something that might create a situation

Drug Free Holistic Approach

where I didn't feel pain in a particular area which would hide the realization that maybe I had a different issue that I needed to work on. So it really was more from a perspective that I was doing medical Qigong exercises which focused on the liver.

In the very first book that I got after getting Parkinson's is entitled What Your Doctor May Not Tell You About Parkinson's Disease by Dr. Jill Marjama-Lyons. It's a really good book because it covers in depth all of the medications that were in place at the time she wrote the book plus it also talks about Traditional Chinese medicine perspective and the Ayurvedic perspective. It is a very, very good book and I would recommend that one to anybody who is new to Parkinson's. I think it covers the gamut from all directions.

From the perspective of traditional

Drug Free Holistic Approach

Chinese medicine perspective one cause of Parkinson's is a liver-wind deficiency. Essentially, a problem with the liver and wind means you shake. My body would have to process any types of medications or supplements through my liver.

I was very much focused on strengthening my liver, cleansing my liver, eating foods that were good for my kidney and liver and really working very hard to cleanse my liver. I sincerely believed in the traditional Chinese medicine view of Parkinson's. Ingesting a medication or a supplement would have been contrary to that philosophy from my point of view. It would have been a little bit counterproductive because it would have made my liver have to work harder in order to process and cleanse my body from medications or supplements.

I feel from my experience that Parkinson's is an electrical problem with the body. It is not a chemical problem. I feel very

Drug Free Holistic Approach

strongly that to recover from Parkinson's you need to deal with it from a neural-electrical impulse perspective, not from taking chemicals that are going to change other chemical balances or imbalances in the body.

> **Why is Parkinson's an electrical problem rather than a chemical problem?**

HOWARD SHIFKE: Even from the way it is viewed clinically, you're not getting the electrical impulses that you're supposed to be getting so movement is impeded. Consider my experience in actually experiencing the disease without medications and without supplements. I would periodically feel pain in an area where I hadn't felt pain or I would periodically have no pain in an area where I felt pain practically all the time. I concluded that the issue is not that the dopamine was dead or even depleted, but rather that dopamine was shut off in some way. It was not able to get all of the electrical impulses to go to where they

Drug Free Holistic Approach

normally needed to go.

I live in Florida so I'll use an example of a hurricane by way of example. After a hurricane comes through and wipes out the electricity for awhile, people put in power generators. Typically the power generator will run your refrigerator and freezer. It will run your air conditioning. It will run the washer and dryer. It will run the lights. But a power generator is not going to run them all at the same time when the electrical company provides a constant flow of electricity to your home. I view the Parkinson's body is analogous to running on a power generator. It isn't that the full ability of the electricity to be there is not there, it is just that somehow it has been cut off.

After they work on the power lines and they get everything fixed and they flip the proper switches, you know you can run everything at the same time: the lights, the air conditioner, the washer, the dryer, the refrigerator and freezer all at the same time. I really feel that Parkinson's follows that same scenario. The body has reached a level where it is working more like on a power generator than on full electricity. The fact that periodically I would feel impulse in places I hadn't felt them for a while made me feel like the nerves weren't dead in those areas and the impulses getting to those areas weren't dead – they just weren't consistent.

Is holistic healing a quick way to recover?

HOWARD SHIFKE: It is a long and difficult way toward recovery, but I will tell you one well worth the fight. I think recovering from any major disease is not going to be quick. Certainly holistic healing is slow because it starts rather deep within. There is a lot of healing that has to take place until you finally get to the surface and really start to see some physical manifestation of recovery.

Drug Free Holistic Approach

> What steps need to be taken to begin a holistic healing program of healing?

HOWARD SHIFKE: When I was about six months into having Parkinson's I started a blog which contains a step-by-step explanation of everything that I did to recover, including all of the resources that were helpful to my recovery. The books and articles that were helpful to me are listed. You will also find five videos of me doing some of the Qi Gong exercises.

The biggest challenge of recovery is having the true belief that you will recover. This is a disease that fights you every minute of every day. The first order of business is starting with the attitude that says, "I will recover," and believing it. I tell people believe it. In order to recover you have to say, "They are incorrect. This is not incurable. I will get better." There is a profound saying by Dr. Sha:

Drug Free Holistic Approach

> *"I have the power to heal myself.*
>
> *You have the power to heal yourself.*
>
> *Together we have the power to heal the world."*

The first and most important step is to believe in your ability to recover from this disease.

I put a lot of focus on the liver and the kidneys and so I did Medical Qi Gong for the liver and the kidneys. I did the exercises every day. A few months after I had started my program of recovery I came across Qi Gong routine for clearing liver-wind. I thought that this routine was incredible because that was really the point of what I was trying to work on.

Standing for any length of time and balance was a terrible challenge for me. There was a standing exercise that I had done for years that I couldn't do anymore

Drug Free Holistic Approach

because I would fall backwards. I actually started standing against the wall. All you do is you stand with this exercise. You bend your knees a little bit. You put your arms up in a way almost like you're holding a beach ball in front of you. And, you just stand there for five minutes–if you can work your way up to five minutes. What this simple exercise does is incredible. You can feel your body strengthening from the inside just by standing.

As we spoke about earlier, I did the awareness of the neural impulses when I was moving one limb at a time and seeing where both limbs were going. I also did the brain-vibration chanting.

When moving during the day I did not feel the tremors much, sometimes not at all. When sitting still and certainly when lying in bed at night the tremors were terrible. There is an acupressure procedure for the nervous system and for Parkinson's. It is

Drug Free Holistic Approach

acupressure of the governing vessel which involves pressing on 20 different pressure points on the body, starting at the coccyx, going up your back and ending at the top of your head.

My wife would do the governing vessel acupressure on me every night. The nightly experience of receiving the governing vessel acupressure treatment helped me really understand that I was dealing with an electrical problem and not a chemical problem. When she would start to do the acupressure at my coccyx in my lower back, I would feel huge surges of electricity shoot down my legs to my feet. As she moved up my back, I could feel electricity moving down to my sides. By the time she finished, I didn't feel tremors. They went away long enough that I could fall asleep.

I know there are people that say that they have a horrific time with Parkinson's and sleeping. I do not recall one bad night of

Drug Free Holistic Approach

sleep. From just dealing with the disease all day I was pretty exhausted at bedtime anyhow. But lying there, experiencing the tremors for the worst of the day because you are just laying there on the bed, the governing vessel acupressure treatment took away the tremors so I could go to sleep. I think that was huge in my recovery.

There's also a modality called <u>Jin Shin Jyutsu</u> which was helpful. It helps balance the energy flows in the body.

I have a book I got on Zen called <u>Not Always So</u>. I would read just one passage every day.

There is a meditation known as sitting <u>Zazen</u>. It is basically meditative sitting. I've never been able to sit in a lotus position, but at least I could sit with my legs crossed. I could not do that for any length of time, so I actually did it sitting in a chair. You sit for ten minutes with your eyes 75% closed, counting your

Drug Free Holistic Approach

breaths from one to ten, and then start over again. It is incredible how relaxing that is. All you are doing is counting your breaths. Instead of trying to clear my mind, my mind cleared itself because all I was doing was focusing on the breaths.

I did along the way adopt a vegetarian diet. One of the things that they say Parkinson's causes is constipation. I had that in a really bad way. By changing to a vegetarian diet I was able to get rid of that problem. From some of the research I had done, I realized that my biggest issue was eating a lot of animal protein during the holidays. When January came around I paid a very bad penalty for that. In January of 2010 I changed to a completely vegetarian diet and have not had a constipation problem since.

A really important and useful website with valuable information I discovered is sponsored by Dr. Janice Walton-Hadlock who has worked with Parkinson's patients

Drug Free Holistic Approach

for about a dozen years - pdrecovery.org. She and her staff work with a modality called the Yin Tui Na, known also as Forceless Spontaneous Release (FSR). It is done using a specialized way of holding a person's foot to help turn around a backward energy flow in the stomach meridian. Dr. Janice Walton-Hadlock discovered along the way that there was a consistency with an old foot or ankle injury that was causing the flow of the stomach meridian to go in the incorrect direction. Opening up that flow facilitates the healing process for Parkinson's. The other side of the formula is the mind part and the soul or heart part of the equation.

I also did a lot of meditation and affirmations and prayers. I worked on getting negative thoughts out of my head. I worked on meditating on positive things. I worked on gratitude meditations. I feel that those were also just as important as all of the physical things that I was doing. I did the physical things because I felt the

Drug Free Holistic Approach

great need to cleanse toxins from my body, re-build the strength of my organs and have my body ready to heal. The meditations and affirmations and prayers really went a long way toward opening up my heart and opening up my mind so that I could recover.

> **Did you see immediate results when you started your program of recovery?**

HOWARD SHIFKE: I did not and I think is the hardest part. It is the getting started with the feeling that someday I will get better. Maybe I won't see any great results right away but I need to stick with this. Holistic healing is not a quick way to recover. It also is not a quick way to feeling great right away.

There were times along the way when I thought, "Okay, I don't think I'm any worse today than I was yesterday." There was a rare occasion here or there where I thought I felt a little better today than I did yesterday. When I went for my three-

Drug Free Holistic Approach

month follow-up visit in February of 2010, my neurologist said he actually was able to detect that my balance seemed better and that my rigidity was probably the same - maybe a tiny bit better. There were some indications that even he could detect but they were very, very small.

> **Why did you stick with holistic healing even though you didn't see any results right away?**

HOWARD SHIFKE: That's the part that takes a lot of faith. The emotional support of family and friends helps. Really it is just a question of concluding that "I need to do this."

Through my blog I communicate with a lot of people. Others have pointed out to me that one of the things that they think probably helped - and I think they are probably correct – is that I have a decade-worth of history doing holistic healing with family members. This helped me know and believe that holistic healing will work. Even though I didn't see

Drug Free Holistic Approach

measurable results right away, I really had a good sense that I would be recovering one day. That's a big part of it.

Conceptually some people feel that they got the disease when they were diagnosed. That would be rare I would guess. Maybe not obvious but it would be very rare. As most people really reflect back, they usually remember: "Wow, I've had some things wrong with me for probably quite some time." Then they realize, "Oh, I have a bigger problem now. I just wasn't paying attention to those little things along the way." You did not get Parkinson's the day you were diagnosed and you're not going to get rid of it the day after the diagnosis.

I imagine that the captain of the Titanic only saw the tip of the iceberg, if even that. History says that an ice mountain had been growing for a long time under the surface. Parkinson's is that way. When the iceberg finally breaks through the surface there is a mountain of layers

Drug Free Holistic Approach

below that need to be dealt with in order to recover. Holistic healing starts from very deep within.

It didn't give me any great feeling on the surface as I was healing my organs. As a matter of fact, I actually lost tactile feeling on the outside of my hand in December of 2009. I couldn't tell the difference between hot water or boiling water. I could cut myself or get a mosquito bite and not feel it. My body had stopped sweating.

Most people find holistic healing to be a difficult concept. More times than not, pain is going to be representative that you're making progress. It is completely turning the general theory of pain on its head. Most of the time we try to avoid pain. We do not want to feel pain. But when you're cleansing toxins with holistic healing they do not leave without a fight.

Holistic healing is something that you have to really be strong-willed about

Drug Free Holistic Approach

because pain is going to be felt. Ultimately that pain is going to go away. I like to refer to it as good pain. If you think about it, what are the consequences when you do a standing exercise. All you are doing is standing. After a couple of minutes of standing, the energy is moving in your body. You start to feel pain. I view that as good pain. There is very little you can do to hurt yourself from a pain perspective by just standing. It takes a bit of a different mindset to really stick with it.

One of the things that helped me stick with it is that I really did not put a lot of worry or concern into when I was going to get better. As a matter of fact I was quite surprised that I had recovered in nine months. I did not have an expectation of that type of result. It was not like I was running in a race. It was more like I was just plodding along. As I tell people sometimes, this is the race won by the tortoise - slow and steady as opposed to the hare – fast and hurried.

Drug Free Holistic Approach

It does take a certain amount of resolve to not become frightened when the disease fights back because it does fight back. If we start a new exercise or start doing something differently and we get some pain with it, the natural thing to do is stop. When we stop it means the disease wins because it gets in your head. It wants you to stop.

I had an argument with myself almost every morning to do the exercises and do the meditation. And face it. I was the one who was taking responsibility for getting better. If I did not do the exercises and I did not do the meditations there would be no possibility of a good ending.

That's one of the things about the disease. I feel very strongly that it just fights you back. I did have a discussion and sometimes an argument with myself: "No. You don't really need to do them. You can skip a day." There is that constant feeling that you have to just keep pushing ahead

Drug Free Holistic Approach

and pushing ahead. At a certain level it's achieving a balance.

As I was progressing along I realized that I did need to work on the meditations. I did need to work on keeping strong faith in those things. If you think about Parkinson's and you think about the soul, mind and body aspect of it, Parkinson's physically knocks you off balance. You move slowly. You have to be more cautious. You are looking down; you are not looking forward. It puts your body in a posture that makes it nearly impossible to walk balanced. With a bent neck and a bent spine and your head looking down, you don't have a good visual frame of reference. You are really out-of-balance physically.

These physical challenges lead to be being knocked off-balance mentally. You become afraid of falling, afraid of freezing, afraid of what people think when they see you, afraid of where the future of

Drug Free Holistic Approach

Parkinson's may take you – a wheelchair or a walker.

That's the thing about Parkinson's. It really knocks everything off-balance. Physically you get knocked off-balance. That leads to mentally getting knocked off-balance. This ultimately leads to spiritually getting knocked off-balance. Facing all of these challenges, one tends to give up hope that you can get better, particularly when you're diagnosed with a disease they tell you cannot get better. It takes a different mindset. Once Parkinson's knocks you off-balance physically, mentally and spiritually, Parkinson's is winning.

Along the way I learned that actually it needed to be flipped around the other way. When I say flipped around the other way, as Dr. Sha would say, "First heal your soul. Your mind and body will follow." It takes a very strong belief and a very strong faith that you have the power to

Drug Free Holistic Approach

heal yourself. You have to know that. Not just think it. You have to know it in your heart. You have to know it in your soul of souls that one day you will get better. I really did. I really felt that way. I was adamant about it. I knew I would get better. I really accepted that as fact.

I knew I needed to have a good attitude and get my mind ready, but on the spiritual side I was really still looking on the outside. And then, really what I needed to do was focus on healing from the inside, from the spiritual side – letting go of my fear of Parkinson's, letting go of negative thoughts about what might happen in the future. Letting go of those types of fears is very liberating in fighting this disease. Fear plays a leading role into making one physically and mentally imbalanced.

The meditations and the affirmations were very, very important. They help reduce adrenaline and open up the doors

Drug Free Holistic Approach

for dopamine. This is an important relationship. Dr. Walton Hadlock writes about the relationship between adrenaline and dopamine which makes very good sense as it relates to Parkinson's.

What happens when you shift into the adrenaline mode? I guess the best example is when you are walking along and a lion jumps out of the bushes and you start running for your life. Your adrenaline kicks in. When you're adrenaline kicks in and you take off, your adrenaline is telling the other parts of your body "I don't want to have to stop for a restaurant break. I'm trying to survive here. I don't want to have to stop and eat or drink because I'm trying to survive here." So I feel that living a fast-paced life and being in the adrenaline mode all the time upsets the balance of the body.

Doing these meditations and doing these affirmations and getting rid of the fear and calming myself and getting rid of the

Drug Free Holistic Approach

anger and things of that nature allowed my adrenaline mode to back off. It allowed the dopamine to flow. I know that this is a theory that many readers just roll their eyes about, but I can tell you sincerely that that is what I experienced.

I actually had a conversation with my adrenaline. I told my adrenaline that for years I needed to be in adrenaline mode just to survive, but all of those stressors in my life that had existed were no longer in existence. It was okay for my adrenaline to back off a little bit.

Then I would have a conversation with my dopamine. I would tell my dopamine:

> *"I know during all of those years that adrenaline was in charge. You had to shut off. You turned the faucet off. Now, my organs aren't functioning properly. My liver isn't functioning properly. My large intestine isn't functioning properly. You did*

Drug Free Holistic Approach

> ***need to get out of the way before, but I need you now."***

The only thing is, I don't know how much of my adrenaline should be backing off and how much of my dopamine should be flowing. What is the proper mix? So I would tell them both:

> ***"I need the two of you to work on this with the Higher Power and I'm going to go meditate on something else so that I don't get in the way of the conversation. But I need to get my body back in the proper flows so that I can get back to being a regular person again and I can recover from this disease."***

Ultimately, I did.

I did my meditations every day. My wife gave me the forceless, spontaneous release (Yin Tui Na) treatments, the foot holding treatments. I would say that I saw

Drug Free Holistic Approach

very, very little results for probably 8 ½ months. After 8 ½ months of seeing very little results I started to see results and they started to happen fast. Within the next two weeks, I was completely symptom-free. That is one of the things about holistic healing. It comes from a place from deep, deep within.

You are doing healing work in areas where you're not aware. How do you know if you're organs are healing? You can't see it. You don't feel it. How do you know if your liver is being cleansed? Those aren't things that you can touch or see or even feel. That's where the faith comes in.

You have to believe in the process, you have to believe that healing is going to happen. If you truly, sincerely believe in the process, then this is where the soul-mind-body connection comes in. When you have faith and you really believe in the process, then your mind doesn't have to worry that it won't work. Your mind will

Drug Free Holistic Approach

follow because if you truly believe you will be successful at some day in the future your mind has no need to worry about any bad consequences. You're working hard with your body and it responds as well. I really feel that Dr. Sha hits the nail on the head when he talks about when healing the soul the mind and body will follow.

Even in that example I gave you about breaking your arm and going to the doctor, if you think about it, when the doctor says, "Robert, your arm is going to be good as new. I'm just going to set it and put it in this cast and then when you come back in x-amount of time, I'll take off the cast and you'll be good as new." If you think about it, you have faith in the doctor and you have faith in the process. The entire time that your arm is in that cast, you don't worry that it isn't going to get better.

What does your body do? It heals itself. It gets better. We never stop and think,

Drug Free Holistic Approach

"Gee, how did this process really work?" Healing happens in my simple example of putting a cast on a broken arm because you believe in the process. You do not grieve over it. I cannot imagine that there are very many children who fall, break their arm, get a cast, are told by the doctor "your arm will be good as new" who fret about the outcome one moment after that. They are back in the playground. They are back outside running around playing. They are not really concerned about it because they have faith in the process. They do not worry about it and they get better. I feel that you can do the same thing with Parkinson's. It's not as easy, but it can have great results.

Can I promise that anybody who does what I did will recover? Of course not. But I have detailed precisely what I did to recover. I have been sharing the information for almost a year now on my blog. I can't see where doing these things

Drug Free Holistic Approach

could have any bad results for anybody. I really feel very strongly that everybody has to get on their own path. The path that I choose - and I notated it very carefully – is repeatable by others. I feel very strongly that others too have a very substantial chance of recovering.

> **Can holistic healing help people who are taking Parkinson's medications?**

HOWARD SHIFKE: I feel that everybody who believes in themselves and believes that their body can heal them should have the opportunity to recover. I don't think that the set of people who are taking Parkinson's medications, which is the greater majority of the people who are diagnosed with Parkinson's, should be negated from the ability to recover. In the grand scheme of life that to me would seem to lack in fairness.

It would be hard for me to imagine that certain lifestyle changes such as adding in some exercises, doing some chanting and

Drug Free Holistic Approach

"Gee, how did this process really work?" Healing happens in my simple example of putting a cast on a broken arm because you believe in the process. You do not grieve over it. I cannot imagine that there are very many children who fall, break their arm, get a cast, are told by the doctor "your arm will be good as new" who fret about the outcome one moment after that. They are back in the playground. They are back outside running around playing. They are not really concerned about it because they have faith in the process. They do not worry about it and they get better. I feel that you can do the same thing with Parkinson's. It's not as easy, but it can have great results.

Can I promise that anybody who does what I did will recover? Of course not. But I have detailed precisely what I did to recover. I have been sharing the information for almost a year now on my blog. I can't see where doing these things

Drug Free Holistic Approach

could have any bad results for anybody. I really feel very strongly that everybody has to get on their own path. The path that I choose - and I notated it very carefully – is repeatable by others. I feel very strongly that others too have a very substantial chance of recovering.

> **Can holistic healing help people who are taking Parkinson's medications?**

HOWARD SHIFKE: I feel that everybody who believes in themselves and believes that their body can heal them should have the opportunity to recover. I don't think that the set of people who are taking Parkinson's medications, which is the greater majority of the people who are diagnosed with Parkinson's, should be negated from the ability to recover. In the grand scheme of life that to me would seem to lack in fairness.

It would be hard for me to imagine that certain lifestyle changes such as adding in some exercises, doing some chanting and

Drug Free Holistic Approach

very, very little results for probably 8 ½ months. After 8 ½ months of seeing very little results I started to see results and they started to happen fast. Within the next two weeks, I was completely symptom-free. That is one of the things about holistic healing. It comes from a place from deep, deep within.

You are doing healing work in areas where you're not aware. How do you know if you're organs are healing? You can't see it. You don't feel it. How do you know if your liver is being cleansed? Those aren't things that you can touch or see or even feel. That's where the faith comes in.

You have to believe in the process, you have to believe that healing is going to happen. If you truly, sincerely believe in the process, then this is where the soul-mind-body connection comes in. When you have faith and you really believe in the process, then your mind doesn't have to worry that it won't work. Your mind will

© *Parkinsons Recovery*   53

Drug Free Holistic Approach

follow because if you truly believe you will be successful at some day in the future your mind has no need to worry about any bad consequences. You're working hard with your body and it responds as well. I really feel that Dr. Sha hits the nail on the head when he talks about when healing the soul the mind and body will follow.

Even in that example I gave you about breaking your arm and going to the doctor, if you think about it, when the doctor says, "Robert, your arm is going to be good as new. I'm just going to set it and put it in this cast and then when you come back in x-amount of time, I'll take off the cast and you'll be good as new." If you think about it, you have faith in the doctor and you have faith in the process. The entire time that your arm is in that cast, you don't worry that it isn't going to get better.

What does your body do? It heals itself. It gets better. We never stop and think,

Drug Free Holistic Approach

meditations and adjusting a dietary strategy would be harmful to somebody. I don't recommend that a person do anything I might recommend without talking to their doctor first in light of the fact that the person and their doctor are the best judges of what is going on in their system based upon the medications that they're taking.

I receive an occasional email from people who are taking medications who saw my blog or watched my videos. They tell me after doing some of these exercises that the outcome has been positive. People have said: "I feel pretty good compared to how I was feeling. I feel a little bit lighter and not as rigid. I have less pain. I feel that my balance is better." I can report that a few people have reported that they have gotten some symptom relief even though they are taking medications.

Many explanations for healing are possible. Doing the exercises that help

Drug Free Holistic Approach

cleanse the liver offer the potential for medications to work better or dosages to be reduced. I would have a hard time seeing harm in doing any of the holistic exercises but every individual is different. The disease affects everybody differently. I would highly recommend before anybody just jump in with both feet that they have a conversation with their doctor about it. I think that that's a really important thing. The doctor is a critical piece of the formula.

What is the address of your blog?

HOWARD SHIFKE: http://www.fightingparkinsonsdrugfree.com

How can people get in touch with you?

HOWARD SHIFKE: My email is: mailto:howard@fightingparkinsonsdrugfree.com. *If you go to the website there's a tab that says "Contact." When you click on that tab, it will bring up the email address as well.*

© *Parkinsons Recovery*

Drug Free Holistic Approach

> **What would you say to someone who has just been diagnosed with Parkinson's disease?**

HOWARD SHIFKE: Don't view it as a death sentence. There are other ways to approach the disease than the conventional methods. Don't give up hope. Don't give up faith. Don't be afraid to share it with at least one other person with whom you are close. I do not believe it is a disease that you should or can fight by yourself. I sincerely believe it is a disease that can fight and you can win. You have the power to heal yourself.

> **How to Hear Howard Shifke on Parkinsons Recovery Radio**

Visit http://www.blogtalkradio.com/parkinsons-recovery and scroll back to find the show that aired March 15, 2011 featuring Howard Shifke as my guest.

> **About Howard Shifke**

I was born in Miami, Florida on March 23, 1961. In 1983, I graduated from college and in 1986, I graduated from

Drug Free Holistic Approach

law school. On October 16, 1988, I married Sally, and we have three wonderful children.

Over the years, I have studied many holistic healing modalities, including Traditional Chinese Medicine, Qigong, Acupressure, Soul, Mind, Body Medicine, Jin Shin Jyutsu, and many meditation techniques. As a result of these healing modalities being successful with health concerns of my family and friends over the years, I grew to have great confidence and faith in their ability to cure disease.

I completely recovered from Parkinson's Disease using a holistic recovery process I designed. It is called my Recipe for Recovery. The Recipe is provided free on my website, <http://www.fightingparkinsonsdrugfree.com>, and also, I offer one-on-one Parkinson's Coaching to assist

Drug Free Holistic Approach

individuals who need help with the Recipe and who wish to gain more in-depth insight into my entire recovery process as I assist them with their recovery.